Coenzyme Q10

All-Around Nutrient for All-Around Health!

Latest research news as a...

HEART STRENGTHENER

ENERGY PROMOTER

AGING FIGHTER

and much more!

A Health Learning Handbook

Beth M. Ley Jacobs, Ph.D.

BL Publications
Temecula, CA

BL Publications, Temecula, CA 92692/ 909-677-1753
health@iinet.com

Ley-Jacobs, Beth M. 1964-
      Coenzyme Q10: all-around nutrient for all-around health!: Latest research as a heart strengthener, energy promoter, aging fighter and much more!/Beth M. Ley Jacobs.
            p.   cm.
      "A Health Learning Handbook"
      Includes bibliographical references and index.
      ISBN: 1-890766-06-2
      1. Ubiquinones--Health aspects.   I. Title.
QP801.U24L49   1999
615'.35--dc21   99-36320
                                                          CIP

Printed in the United States of America

First edition, August 1999
Second edition, October 1999

This book is not intended as medical advice. It's purpose is solely educational. Always consult your medical physician for any medical situation.

This book does not support any specific manufacturer, brand or supplemental form of CoQ10. The information provided is for your reference so you can make your own decision on what is best for your needs.

Credits:
Typesetting and Cover Design: BL Publications
Research and Technical Assistance: Richard Conant
Proofreading: Michelle Warnes, Virginia Simpson-Magruder

Table of Contents

Health Learning Handbooks

These books are designed to provide useful information about ways to improve one's health and well-being. Education about what the body needs to obtain and maintain good health is what we would like to provide.

Good health should not be thought of as absence of disease. We should avoid negative disease-oriented thinking and concentrate on what we have to do to remain healthy. Health is maintaining on a daily basis what is essential to the body. Disease is the result of attempting to live without what the body needs. We are responsible for our own health and should take control of it. If we are in control of our health, disease is not likely to take control.

Our health depends on education.

Books in this series include:

Aspirin Alternatives: Top Natural Pain-Relieving Analgesics by Raymond Lombardi, D.C., N.D., C.C.N.

Castor Oil: Its Healing Properties by Beth Ley

CoQ10: All-Around Nutrient for All-Around Health by Beth Ley Jacobs, Ph.D.

Dr. John Willard on Catalyst Altered Water by Beth Ley

Colostrum: Nature's Gift to the Immune System by Beth Ley

DHA: The Magnificent Marine Oil by Beth Ley Jacobs

How to Fight Osteoporosis and Win! The Miracle of Microcrystalline Hydroxyapatite by Beth Ley

PhytoNutrients: Medicinal Nutrients Found in Foods by Beth Ley

MSM: On Our Way Back to Health with Sulfur by Beth Ley

Nature's Road to Recovery: Nutritional Supplements for the Alcoholic and Chemical-Dependent by Beth Ley Jacobs, Ph.D.

The Potato Antioxidant: Alpha Lipoic Acid by Beth Ley

The True Vitamin C: Mineral Ascorbates! by Beth Ley Jacobs, Ph.D.

For order information, see page 70.

Introduction

Coenzyme Q10: Your Time Has Come!

Many supplements that have been in existence for sometimes decades or longer, eventually reach a time where they finally "make it!" Recent examples of supplements finally getting the acceptance they deserve include DHEA, pregnenolone, colostrum, MSM, glucosamine, and lipoic acid.

Coenzyme Q10 (CoQ10) is a naturally occurring substance that has properties potentially beneficial for the entire body. It is especially well-known for its ability to prevent cellular damage during and following a heart attack (myocardial ischemia and reperfusion). Orally it is used therapeutically in the treatment of various cardiovascular disorders, including angina pectoris, hypertension, high blood cholesterol and congestive heart failure. It is also used in the treatment of periodontal disease, immune deficiency, diabetes, AIDS and the various mitochondrial diseases. These will be discussed in more detail later.

A Brief History

- In 1957, Dr. Frederick Crane of Wisconsin isolated an orange substance from the mitochondria of beef heart.

- In 1958, Dr. Karl Folkers (who is often recognized as the "Father of CoQ10 Research") and co-workers at Merck, Sharpe and Dohme were able to determine the exact chemical structure and synthesize CoQ10 in a laboratory.

- In the 1960's, Japanese researcher, Dr. Tora

Yamamura, successfully used CoQ7 in the therapy of congestive heart failure.

● In 1972, Dr. Folkers and Italian researcher, Dr. Littarru, documented a CoQ10 deficiency in human heart disease. Also in the 1970s, researchers discovered that CoQIO has antioxidant abilities.

● In 1974, Japanese scientists perfected the industrial technology to produce sufficient CoQ10 for distribution.

● In 1978, English researcher, Peter Mitchell, received a Nobel Prize for CoQ10 and energy transfer.

● In the 1980's, CoQ10 scientific research increased around the world.

● In 1987, *The Miracle Nutrient Coenzyme Q10* by Emile Bliznakov and Gerald Hunt (Bantam Books), introduced CoQ10 to the general public.

● In the 1990's, CoQ10 gained popularity in the health food industry.

The majority of people (including many doctors), unfortunately, have never heard of CoQ10. Hopefully, this book will help change that. Many doctors in Europe are already prescribing CoQ10 to patients with congestive heart failure. In Japan since the late1970s, CoQ10 has been widely accepted as a preventative and treatment for those with heart disease. Since 1982, CoQ10 consumption has rivaled the country's top five medications. For years, the Japanese led the world in research on this amazing nutrient.

Since 1976, there have been 10 international symposiums on the biochemical and clinical benefits of CoQ10. This includes over 350 scientific papers presented by over 200 different physicians and researchers from 18 different countries who have examined CoQ10 supplementation in a wide range of medical disorders. The evidence is overwhelming!

CoQ10:
The All-Around Nutrient

CoQ10's chemical structure is 2,3 dimethoxy-5 methyl-6 decaprenyl benzoquinone. It is also known as ubiquinone. The name was formed from the word **ubiquitous** *(which Websters defines as "existing or being present everywhere at the same time")* and the coenzyme **quinone**, because Coenzyme Q is found in virtually every cell in the body.

CoQ10 has a molecular structure similar to Vitamin K and could be considered a relative of Vitamin E. It is found in humans, animals, and plants. In plants it is known as plastoquinone. Animals and humans have a variety of molecular formulations ranging from CoQ6 to CoQ10. The numbered designation refers to the number of isoprene units in the molecular chain. CoQ6 to Co10 are found in animals, while only CoQ10 is found in humans. Although CoQ10 is the form utilized by the body for energy, Q6—9 can be changed into Q10 when ingested as part of the diet.

While CoQ10 is found in virtually every cell in the body, its concentration varies depending on the tissue type and location. The heart tissue contains more CoQ10 than any other organ in the body. Therefore, CoQ10 deficiencies are likely to first affect the heart. However, effects may be seen anywhere CoQ10 is needed. This could be in any organ, tissue or system in the body — the brain, kidneys, lungs, pancreas, periodontal tissues, immune system, etc.

If the body is low or deficient in CoQ10, supplementing CoQ10 is likely to be beneficial having a wide range of variable effects depending upon the individual.

CoQ10 Tissue Concentrations

	mcg/gram
Heart	114.0
Kidney	66.5
Liver	54.9
Pancreas	32.7
Brain	13.4
Colon	10.7 (Ernster)

Organs such as the heart and liver that require the largest supplies of energy to function have high concentrations of CoQ10. Heart muscle and neurons (nerve cells such as in the brain or central nervous system) have the greatest concentration of mitochondria—as many as 5,000 per cell.

Levels of CoQ10 in the body are influenced by factors such as age. stress, cold, illness, hormone concentrations, drugs and physical activity. Reduced levels may lead to reduced energy and reduced functioning of any organ or gland in the body. After the age of 20, humans experience a gradual decline in CoQ10 levels.

CoQ10 deficiency may be caused by insufficient dietary CoQ10, impairment in CoQ10 biosynthesis, excessive utilization of CoQ10 by the body, use of certain medications - especially STATINS, which are cholesterol reducing drugs, or any combination of these.

Factors That Lower CoQ10 Levels:

- **Certain Medications (especially "STATINS")**
- **Age**

- **Alcohol Consumption**
- **Nutrient Status: Vitamin B-6, Selenium, etc.**
- **Strenuous Exercise** (Kaikkonen)
- **Other Stressors: Extreme Cold, Illness, etc.**

Some Drugs Lower CoQ10 Levels

Many drugs adversely affect the production of CoQ10 in the body, and supplementation with CoQ10 can reduce the adverse effects associated with these medications. Examples include Lovastatin (Diebold, Mortensen), (which is commonly used to lower cholesterol), and beta-blockers (which help decrease blood pressure). In some cases, long-term use of beta-blockers has led to congestive heart failure. The CoQ10 lowering effects of these medications seem to be more prominent in older individuals. The effects are also dose related and researchers are now recommending CoQ10 supplementation for individuals on long-term therapy of these medications. (Mortensen)

Common psychotropics (drugs that modify mood or behavior), such as antidepressants, also inhibit CoQ10-dependent enzymes. CoQ10 supplementation may help prevent some of the side effects of these medications.

How CoQ10 Works

There are two basic functions which CoQ10 provides in the body.

• **Provides Energy:** CoQ10 transports electrons involved in energy metabolism within the mitochondria inside each of our cells.

• **Provides Antioxidant Protection:** CoQ10 is a very powerful antioxidant against free radicals, which cause or contribute to many various degenerative diseases. It is just as important as Vitamins E and C.

1. Provides Energy

The mitochondria is the part of each cell which produces energy (ATP) that is needed for the functioning of each cell and the life of the entire body. CoQ10 is essential for the production of adenosine 5 triphosphate (ATP), and thus is present in all tissues of the body.

Succinate dehydrogenase-co-Q-10 reductase is the enzyme needed for the production of ATP. The calories from the food (amino acids, sugars and fats) we eat is extracted to build more ATP.

Molecules are composed of atoms held together by bonds. It is the breaking of the ATP molecule's bonds that releases energy. A considerable amount of energy is stored in the bonds that link the two outermost phosphate groups with the remainder of the ATP molecule. When the outermost bond is broken, it releases energy equivalent to about 7,000 calories.

Enzymes are protein substances found in all living things. They are necessary for the building and rebuilding of tissues and cells. Enzymes are catalysts that influence all life systems. They are produced by living cells but are capable of acting independently. Enzymes are specific in their action; they will act only on a certain substance or a group of closely related substances and no others.

Enzymes are made of at least two parts: the protein part and the cofactor part. Genetics determine the specific amino acids that make up the protein portion. Mineral ions (such as calcium, magnesium and zinc) or vitamins, or both, make up the cofactor portion. The vitamin portion is usually called the coenzyme.

The human body must continuously be supplied with its own form of energy to perform its many complex operations. Only enough ATP is stored in the body to provide

---

Mitochondrial Problems

The mitochondria are subject to a lot of free radical damge. When electrons from sugar and fat are combined with oxygen in the manufacture of ATP, reactive and potentially destructive forms of oxygen, known as free radicals, are formed inside the mitochondria. Free radicals are normally neutralized by a specialized enzyme present throughout the mitochondria, known as superoxide dismutase (SOD). Without adequate supplies of SOD, free radicals can roam the cell and damage the mitochondria and other structures.

This type of damage may be the cause of numerous mitochondrial diseases (see page 42-48) and seems to be the explanation for the destruction of motor neurons in ALS, or Lou Gehrig's disease, a usually fatal paralytic disease.

---

energy to sustain strenuous activity for 5 to 8 seconds. Aside from the energy needed for work performed by the muscular system, there is a considerable demand for energy by other biological systems. This includes the energy for digestion, absorption and assimilation of the food nutrients. This energy is also needed for the functioning of various endocrine glands, for the establishment of the proper muscle status, for circulation, cardiovascular health, blood pressure, the immune system, etc.

CoQ10 is the key to the process that produces 95% of cellular energy. The foods we eat and store in ready access within the body provide the basic raw material to change into ATP with the help of CoQ10. The body extracts the potential energy stored within the structure of carbohydrate, fat and protein molecules consumed in the diet or stored in the body. This energy is harnessed for one major purpose, to combine adenosine and phosphate to form the energy-rich compound ATP.

2. Provides Antioxidant Protection

CoQ10 is a powerful antioxidant from which the entire body and entire array of body systems can benefit.

- The cardiovascular system and the heart itself

- The circulatory system—preventing free radical damage throughout the entire body

- The immune system—improving the body's ability to cope with free radicals

- The metabolic system—aiding with energy production and also assisting with weight control.

Over 80 diseases and health problems are associated with free radical damage. These include:

Allergies	Kidney disease
Alzheimer's disease	Liver disease
Arthritis	Lupus
Asthma	Neuropathy
Cancer	Macular degeneration
Cataracts	Parkinson's disease
Cardiovascular disease	Psoriasis
Diabetes	Premature aging
Gingivitis	Senile dementia
Hemorrhoids	Varicose veins
HIV	Vascular weakness (bruise easily)
Huntington's disease	Wrinkles
Impaired immune function	

Consumed regularly, CoQ10 fights off the aging process as it contributes to greater health and longevity. CoQ10 provides valuable protection from oxidative damage occurring in fat-soluble media such as cell membranes, which are composed of fatty acids. It also works with Vitamin E to prevent damage to lipid membranes and plasma lipids. Like other antioxidants, CoQ10 also offers protection against the accumulation and deposit of oxidized fats in blood vessels, which can lead to atherosclerosis (Weber, Thomas, Alleva).

CoQ10 is believed to be the first antioxidant to be depleted when LDL is faced with oxidation. (Stocker) In the bloodstream, CoQ10 is mainly transported by lipoproteins, such as low-density lipoproteins (LDL) and high-density lipoproteins (HDL). CoQ10 is an extremely important nutrient that prevents the lipid peroxidation of lipoproteins. This is how it protects our arteries from plaque formation and other damage.

The effectiveness of antioxidants to protect us against oxidative stress depends on their reactivity towards the oxidative stress depends on their reactivity towards the specific free radical molecules. It is best to have adequate levels of the various intracellular antioxidants such as Vitamins C (ascorbate) and E and lipoic acid. Also very important are the antioxidant enzymes or intermediates of electron transport (such as CoQ10), which also recycle other antioxidants, thus enhancing overall antioxidant protection. (Kagan)

CoQ10 and Vitamin E Protect LDL Cholesterol from Oxidation

LDL oxidation is a process implicated as one of the contributing factors in atherogenesis (heart disease). Australian researchers investigated the effects of supplementation with Vitamin E alone or in combination with CoQ10 against the early stages of oxidation of isolated LDL.

They found that LDL was markedly more resistant to initiation of oxidation with cosupplementation of both Vitamin E and CoQ10 compared to supplementation of Vitamin E alone. (Thomas)

Other researchers have also documented the antioxidant benefits and protective effects from CoQ10 supplementation on LDL peroxidation. Italian researchers specifically demonstrated that a dense subfraction of LDL, namely LDL3, commonly regarded as the most peroxidizable and atherogenic type of LDL, was at a reduced risk for peroxidation after CoQ10 supplementation.

Distribution of CoQ10 among different classes of

CoQ10 helps prevent free radical damage from LDL cholesterol!

14

plasma lipoproteins was also studied: They found about 60% of plasma CoQ10 was associated with LDL. (Alleva)

CoQ10 and Aging

While the average life expectancy is around 80 years, our life potential is believed to be at least 120 years, and may be as high as 140 years. As knowledge increases the potential for major changes in the length of survival of humans increases as well.

Aging is a complex biological process associated with a progressive decline in the physiological and biochemical performance of individual tissues and organs. This decline leads to age-associated diseases and aging.

In keeping with the free radical theory of aging, the antioxidant properties of CoQ10 have clear implications in the slowing of aging and age related degenerative diseases.

Lowered blood and tissue levels of CoQ10 have been observed in a number of clinical conditions. Many of these clinical conditions are most prevalent among the elderly. Studies have shown that blood levels of CoQ10 decline with age (Kalen) and researchers have demonstrated that CoQ10 deficiencies are more prevalent with age. We may lose our ability to produce CoQ10 from other coQ's we obtain from food. It is also suggested that the cells may demand more than we can produce. As health problems (such as heart disease or cancer) become more prevalent with age, higher amounts of CoQ10 may be needed as well.

Free radicals play a major role in the aging process. A therapy designed to prevent free radical damage (called redox therapy) based on CoQ10 supplementation demonstrates profound improvement in heart function of old rats, while no significant effect was observed with young rats (assumed to have normal CoQ10 levels). (Linnane)

Nutrient Status

CoQ10 is found in small amounts in a wide variety of foods, but authorities such as the late Dr. Karl Folkers, believe that this is not our primary source for the body. CoQ10 is synthesized in all tissues of the body. The biosynthesis of CoQ10 from the amino acid tyrosine is a multistage process requiring at least eight vitamins and several trace elements. These include taurine, tyrosine, methionine, Vitamins C, B-5, B-6, B-12, folate, and selenium. If deficiencies of any of these nutrients is present, the production level of CoQ10 could be significantly reduced.

Vitamin B-6: Biosynthesis of CoQ10 from tyrosine is dependent on adequate Vitamin B-6 levels in the body. Natural sources of Vitamin B-6 include: Brewer's yeast, bananas, avocados, wheat germ, leafy green vegetables, whole grains and cereals, bananas, milk, eggs, blackstrap molasses, cabbage, soybeans, walnuts, peanuts and pecans. ***Note:*** Vitamin B-6 supplements should not be used by individuals with Parkinson's taking L-dopa.

Vitamin B-6 levels also decline with age. (Kant) Studies are currently in progress to determine the effects of supplementation with Vitamin B-6 on blood CoQ10 levels. It appears that individuals supplementing CoQ10 should also supplement Vitamin B-6 to provide for better endogenous synthesis of CoQ10 (which occurs in the body) along with the exogenous CoQ10 (which we get obtain from the foods we eat). (Willis and Folkers)

Selenium: Selenium, a trace mineral and antioxidant, plays an important role in the production of CoQ10 (and also another energy-producing enzyme, glutathione peroxidase). Low levels of selenium result in a deficiency of CoQ10. If you do not have enough selenium, which is also an antioxidant, to maintain adequate CoQ10 levels, a undesirable cycle of oxidation can result. If CoQ10 is missing from the the energy chain, free radical production is much more likely to occur, for there is a missing link in the energy process. (Null)

Selenium is found in many foods, but the amount is dependent upon the richness and health of the soil in which the food was grown. Food sources of selenium include brewer's yeast, organ and muscle meats, fish and shellfish, grains, cereals and dairy products.

Note: Selenium is one of the most potentially toxic nutrients. Some experts believe that supplementing amounts higher than 400 mcg. daily should be avoided. The standard suggested daily supplemental intake is 200 mcg.

L-Carnitine: This amino acid may be very helpful for many of the conditions for which COQ10 is beneficial. Stephen Sinatra, M.D., author of *The Coenzyme Q10 Phenomenon,* states he often prescribes one to three grams of L-carnitine if the therapeutic response of CoQ10 supplementation is not significant. (Sinatra)

Sources of CoQ10

The body makes CoQ10 from the amino acids tyrosine and methionine. While CoQ10 is available from food sources, we do not always consume enough of these foods to meet the needs of the body. The therapeutic amounts needed far exceed what the body can make or absorb from food.

CoQ10 is found in various foods such as beans, beef, eggs, fish (especially codfish, mackerel, salmon, sardines) and fish oil, spinach, whole grains and the germs of whole grains, vegetable oils and organ meats. These are also the best sources of Vitamin E, which synergistically enhances CoQ10's effects.

Following are examples of the CoQ10 content found in foods:

Fish

Sardine	6.43
Mackerel	4.33
Yellow tail	2.07

Meat

Organ meats	4.0
Beef	3.18
Pork	2.43-4.11
Chicken	2.18

Nuts and Seeds

Peanuts (roasted)	2.67
Sesame seeds (roasted)	2.30
Pistachios (roasted)	2.01
Walnuts (raw)	1.90
Hazelnuts (raw)	1.70
Sweet almonds (roasted)	1.38

Dairy products

Butter	0.71
Eggs	0.37
Cheese	0.21
Cow's milk	0.04

Oils

Soybean oil	9.23
Corn oil	1.30
Sunflower oil	0.42
Safflower oil	0.40
Olive oil	0.41

Cereals

Soybeans (whole/dry)	0.3 - 1.9
Rice bran	0.49
Wheat germ	0.35
Buckwheat	0.11

Vegetables

Spinach	1.02
Broccoli	0.86
Sweet peppers	0.33
Sweet potato	0.36
Garlic	0.27
Carrot	0.22
Eggplant	0.21
Cabbage	0.16
Cauliflower	0.14
Onion	0.10
Potato	0.10

NOTE: *When any of these foods are cooked over 50 degrees Celsius (122 degrees Fahrenheit), the Q10 content is totally destroyed. The Q10 content is highest in raw, fresh foods and diminishes rapidly as freshness is lost in a matter of days.*

To put dietary CoQ10 intake into perspective, one pound of sardines, two pounds of beef, or two and one half pounds of peanuts, provide 30 mg. of CoQ10. Typical dietary intake of CoQ10 can range from 0 to around 20 mg. per day. Meat eaters may have a higher consumption than non-meat eaters. (Hallstrom)

Few people eat enough of the foods providing significant amounts of CoQ10 daily to replenish their supply. Food that has been processed provides little or no CoQ10 (or CoQ9 which can be converted to CoQ10).

Unfortunately, the body's ability to synthesize the CoQ10 from food sources declines with age. So, without supplementation, older individuals can readily develop CoQ10 deficiencies. By age 40, many of us can expect some level of deficiency. Substantial research demonstrates a strong correlation between this CoQ10 deficiency and various problems which can range from lack of energy, to heart disease, to major ill health.

Attention: Vegetarians

Because many of the food sources of CoQ10 are animal based, some authorities believe that strict vegetarians may not be obtaining optimal amounts. Vegetarians may consider increasing consumption of unprocessed soy and peanut products or supplementing a low dosage of CoQ10 to ensure optimal CoQ10 levels in the body.

Supplemental Forms

CoQ10 originally extracted from beef heart for supplemental purposes, was not commercially feasible because of the high expense in doing so. In the 1970's the Japanese developed a fermentation process that has provided mass-production and affordable prices for CoQ10.

CoQ10 is a relatively large, fat-soluble molecule with variable absorption into the body. Oral CoQ10 is now available in tablets, capsules, softgels containing an oil-base suspension, and a hydrosoluble form, known as QGel®.

Some sources claim that bioavailability of dry-form CoQ10 capsules (which is usually the most economical form) can be enhanced by taking it with some fat-containing food or emptying the contents into a tablespoon containing small amount of oil such as sesame, olive or flax. Jarrow Formulas of Los Angeles, Ca, has demonstrated that their Q-Sorb™ CoQ10, a proliposome lipid soluble delivery system increases CoQ10 levels in humans at least 28% higher than dry capsules.

Manufactures have also developed a number of additional ways to enhance absorption.

Bioperine® Increases CoQ10 Bioavailability

Bioperine® (peperine) is a purified alkaloid derived from black pepper, which is commonly used in Ayurvedic medicine to enhance digestion of other foods and medicines. A study has shown that when Bioperine® is combined with CoQ10, bioavailability is enhanced compared to CoQ10 ingested without Bioperine®.

A double-blind study conducted by the manufacturer of Bioperine®, Sabinsa Corporation, Piscataway, NJ (723-777-1111), administered 120 mg. CoQ10 in a softgel supplement to healthy males for 21 days. Another group of males were given 120 mg. CoQ10 together with 5 mg. Bioperine® for 21 days. The results were as follows: (Badmaev)

CoQ10 Alone	CoQ10 w/ Bioperine®

	CoQ10 Alone	CoQ10 w/ Bioperine®
Increase in blood serum over base	0.85 ug./ml.	1.12 ug./ml.

The following is a testimony from a user of CoQ10 with Bioperine® courtesy of Doctor's Best. Inc. For more information, call 1-800-333-6977.

"I wanted to tell you how good Doctor's Best High Absorption Co-Q10 is. This vitamin is the best. I've taken it since 1991.

My son-in-law's vitamin doctor and my daughter were talking about my heart condition. He told her that Co-Q10 would help me breathe better, which it has. Now I take 180 mg. with other vitamins every day, Co-Q10 helps me with oxygen and I'm not so short of breath. I also take Chelation. I hardly have any angina pains. I threw my patches away. I think it's wonderful.

Thanks, Ruth

P.S. If everyone would write me I would write and tell them about Co-Q10."

The manufacturers of CoQsol, Soft Gel Technologies (SGTI™), (1-800-360-7484), report they have conducted randomized, double blind placebo controlled intestinal absorption studies to show their oil soluble capsules have a delivery system almost 3 times as effective as other formulations.* The results showed that a single 30 mg dose of CoQsol, increased the blood CoQ10 level to 2.7 ug./ml. compared to 1.7 ug./ml. for those taking the dry formulation.

Research conducted by the manufacturer of Q-Gel®, a proprietary water-solubilized form, Tishcon Corp. (1-800-848-8442), claims that Q-Gel® has a higher dissolution compared to regular softgels, tablets, and capsules, and also produces higher absorption in the body. In their research they state that after 3 weeks of supplementing 120 mg. Q-Gel®/day, relative mean serum CoQ10 values were two to three times higher compared to levels from the other forms tested.* (Chopra)

(*Note: CoQ10 with Bioperine® was not included in the comparisons.)

Topical or Transdermal CoQ10

Excessive exposure to UV rays can overwhelm the naturally occurring antioxidant capacity of the skin. This can lead to free radical damage and ultimately to skin cancer, immunosuppression and premature skin aging (wrinkles, brown spots, etc.). Transdermal delivery (application to the skin through creams, patches, etc.) of various antioxidants, such as glutathione, catalase, superoxide dismutase (SOD), Vitamin E, ascorbate (Vitamin C) and beta-carotene (pro-Vitamin A) have shown to be very effective in protecting the skin from free radical damaged caused by UVA rays from the sun. (Steenvoorden) A number of manufacturers have released "anti-aging, anti-wrinkle" creams, lotions, etc., containing antioxidants.

CoQ10 is also part of the body's naturally occurring endogenous antioxidant protective system. A recent study at the Paul Gerson Unna Skin Research Center in Hamburg, Germany, with CoQ10 applied transdermally to the skin surface showed CoQ10 did penetrate into the epidermis and dermis layers of the skin and was able to reduce wrinkles by reducing oxidative stress against UVA.

The researchers concluded that CoQ10 is suitable for use in cosmetics and has the potential to prevent many of the detrimental effects of photoaging. (Hoppe)

At least one mass market manufacture has released two separate "wrinkle control" products containing CoQ10 and other antioxidants and there will be more in the near future as the awareness and popularity of CoQ10 increases.

Local application of CoQ10 to the gum tissues improves periodontal symptoms. Topical applications of CoQ10 appears to reduce bleeding and the depth of pockets formed around teeth by receding gums. (Hanioka)

Side Effects/Warnings

Because CoQ10 is a naturally-occurring substance found in the body, and because we do obtain small amounts of it from the foods we eat, the risk of side effects from supplementation is very low.

The side effects that have been reported are very mild and only occurred in 1.5% of individuals with congestive heart failure taking 100 mg. daily for 3 months. (Baggio) Long-term use at even high dosages (over 600 mg. daily) is considered to be very safe. (Greenberg, Feigin)

Some people report that CoQ10 increases energy levels, so you may consider taking your supplement in the morning so not to interfere with sleep at night. Sleep difficulties have been reported by a few individuals using CoQ10 at bedtime. While a small number of individuals have reported that even a low dose (10 mg.) gives them a jittery feeling, this can be reduced by taking CoQ10 with food.

Side effects reported in a study at Mt. Sinai Hospital and Medical Center, New York, with 5,000 people when taking CoQ10 include: *Stomach discomfort*: 19 people; *Loss of appetite:* 11 people; *Mild nausea:* 8 people; *Diarrhea*: 6 people. (Greenberg)

Again, these side effects can be diminished by taking CoQ10 with a meal, preferably in the morning.

Note: It is important to point out that these side effects (and others) are commonly experienced by individuals only taking a placebo. Do not let these stop you from trying CoQ10 for yourself so you can make your own decision whether it is right for you.

While CoQ10 should be safe for pregnant or lactating women, it is wise to consult a physician before use as there is not a great deal of research data in this area. There is some data on high risk pregnancies (spontaneous abortions, complications, etc.) in women who had low CoQ10 levels. (Noria) More research needs to be done before recommendations can be made.

Dosages

CoQ10 deficiencies can be determined through blood levels obtained through your nutrition-oriented physician. Healthy average blood levels for CoQ10 should be in the range of 0.5-0.9 mcg./ml. If you are below this level, you may greatly benefit from CoQ10 supplementation.

Appropriates dosages will depend on the delivery system you select (capsules, oil-based capsules, Q-Gel®, CoQSol®, or other forms), the level of deficiency, dietary habits and various other factors. General starting dosage guidelines for dry-form capsules are as follows:

- **Anti-aging/preventative:**
    30 to 50 mg. daily

- **Cardiovascular /gum disease preventative:**
    75 to150 mg. daily

- **Treatment for atherosclerosis, high blood pressure, diabetes, gum disease, etc.:**
    125 to 300 mg. daily *

- **Treatment for congestive heart failure, cancer, HIV, and other severe immune deficiency:**
    300 to 450 mg. daily *

- **Treatment for Parkinson's, Huntington's and other neurological disorders:**
    As high as 600 to 1,200 mg. daily *

*Maintenance dosages may be lower after improved well-being is achieved.

"Degenerative diseases like Alzheimer's, Parkinson's and Huntington's disease also have defects in energy production, so Coenzyme Q-10 could be important."

Professor Lester Packer at the University of California, Berkeley

CoQ10 and a Healthy Heart

Frank, a 59 year old male, was taking antihypertensive medication for his high blood pressure. He had been diagnosed with coronary artery disease. He easily became out of breath and occasionally experienced a chest tightness that concerned him. He began taking 60 mg. CoQ10 twice daily. After 8 weeks not only was his blood pressure reduced, he also experienced a reduction in triglycerides, fasting insulin and glucose levels,and lipid peroxides (damaging free radicals created by oxidation of fatty acids). His HDL cholesterol (the "good" one) level increased and his levels of antioxidants (Vitamins A, C, E and beta carotene) all increased, suggesting a reduction in oxidative stress. He felt better, had more energy and improved breathing and reduced chest tightness.

This is just one story demonstrating the typical benefits experienced by someone with heart problems who starts taking CoQ10.

Karl Folkers, Ph.D., the world's leading researcher of CoQ10, was awarded the Priestley Medal, the American Chemical Society's most prestigious honor, for his landmark CoQ1O research. In accepting his award he praised CoQ10 as a momentous contributor to human health and especially for its benefits for the heart. Dr. Folkers lived to be more than 90 years old and was an example of the benefits of CoQ10, which he consumed the last 40 years of his life.

Folkers, in his Priestley Medal Address, focused on the dramatic effects he had personally observed and demonstrated through his research, especially among individuals with advanced cardiac disease.

Because heart requires so much CoQ10, many of CoQ10's supplemental beneficial effects are on the heart. The heart requires the largest supply of energy compared to other organs in the body. The heart muscle never stops. In order for us to maintain life, the heart must continue to pump blood, which requires energy and CoQ10.

Folkers' research has shown that blood and tissue concentrations of CoQ10 were significantly lower in heart-disease patients than in those who were heart-disease free.

Research by eminent heart surgeon, Denton Cooley, M.D., confirmed Folkers' findings in that biopsies of 75% of cardiac patients had varying, but significant, deficiencies of CoQ10 in the heart. Folkers reviewed clinical reports by 110 Japanese cardiac specialists in which CoQ10 was given to thousands of patients with heart problems between the years of 1967 and 1976. Two of the large research projects were double-blind studies.

As an effective free radical scavenger, CoQ10 reduces oxidative damage to the heart and thereby reduces the risk of subsequent coronary artery disease.

CoQ10 is particularly useful for patients undergoing heart surgery. Return of blood flow (reperfusion) after surgery results in oxidative damage to the vascular endothelium (cells that line body cavities such as the heart) and myocardium (middle layer of the heart walls). Surgery also depletes naturally occurring levels of CoQ10. Numerous animal and human studies have shown that pre- and post-treatment with CoQ10 can significantly improve treatment outcomes, speed recovery time and protect heart arteries and muscle from subsequent oxidative damage resulting from ischemic and reperfusion injury.

One double-blind, placebo-controlled trial found a significant reduction in cardiac symptoms in individuals receiving oral treatment with CoQ10 (120 mg/day) compared to a placebo group. After 28 days of treatment, the following **reductions** were seen in the following cardiac events:

	Placebo	**CoQ10 Group**
Angina pectoris	9.5 %	28.1 %
Total arrhythmias	9.5 %	25.3 %
Poor left ventricular function	8.2 %	22.5 %
Deaths/nonfatal infarction	15.0 %	30.9 %

Antioxidants Vitamin A, E, C and beta-carotene, which were lower initially in patients after they experienced a major heart attack, increased more in the CoQ10 group than in the placebo group. The researchers suggested that CoQ10 can provide rapid protective effects in heart attack patients if it is administered within 3 days. (Singh)

"I use Doctor's Best CoQ10 (with Bioperine®), which has just about eliminated the episodes of irregular heartbeat I had been experiencing due to Mitral Valve Prolapse."
Nancy

Beneficial for Congestive Heart Failure

Congestive heart failure (CHF) is a condition involving a weak or energy-starved heart. Cells require oxygen to produce energy. Our heart is made of muscle tissue. This muscle weakens with time, aging, poor diet, heart attacks, stress, viral infections, smoking, and alcohol abuse.

As the heart pumps less efficiently, blood and fluid can slowly back up into the lungs and the rest of the body, leading to congestive heart failure. The backup of fluid into the lungs is called pulmonary edema; fluid in the lower extremities is called peripheral edema.

Drugs such as digitalis, a heart stimulant derived from the purple foxglove plant, and diuretics, which drain off excess body fluids through the urine, have been largely unsuccessful in managing congestive heart failure.

By increasing cellular energy, CoQ10 has a direct beneficial effect on the energy-depleted heart muscle. Researchers have demonstrated a significant recovery of cellular oxygen consumption and an "appreciable recovery of" the heart's energy-producing ability.

Energy-boosting and cardiostimulatory effects were pointed out by Dr. Kishi and colleagues, who found increases in cellular ATP production with CoQ10 supplementation.

Dr. Folkers has shown that 70% of heart patients with congestive heart failure benefited from taking CoQ10. After giving 100 mg. of CoQ10 daily to 28 patients with congestive heart failure, Jack H. Hall, M.D., of Methodist Hospital of Indiana, Indianapolis, found a definite improvement of heart function in every case, with no side effects.

Within a month of taking 100 mg. of CoQ10 daily, eight of 12 patients with congestive heart failure who had failed to respond to digitalis and diuretics showed significant improvements.

In 1993, Italian researchers, examined 2,500 patients with congestive heart failure at 173 sites and institutions. Preliminary results with 1,113 patients showed that those who received CoQ10 supplementation as an adjunct to regular treatment experienced improvements in 12 cardiac indicators, from 49.3 to 82.4%.

Another clinical trial on the treatment of chronic cardiac insufficiency with CoQ10 revealed significant improvements in several important cardiac parameters such as ejection fraction, stroke volume, cardiac output, cardiac index and end diastolic volume index. The researchers suggested a CoQ10 daily dosage of 100-200 mg. (Soja)

CoQ10 can also inhibit clotting, which may be one of the mechanisms by which it improves cardiovascular functioning in chronic heart failure.

An additional nutrient to consider among individuals with congestive heart failure is L-carnitine, at one to three grams per day. This nutrient helps transport long-chain fatty acids across the mitochondrial membrane and promotes energy production.

COQ10 Reduces Angina!

Individuals with ischemic heart disease suffer from reduced blood supply to the myocardium, the vascularized muscle layer of the heart wall. This decreases the oxygen supply to the heart, sometimes causing reduced heart function. This can be caused by arterial embolisms, or blood clots in arteries that feed the heart with oxygen-carrying blood, and atherosclerosis, the narrowing of heart arteries caused by plaque buildup.

Reduced oxygen supply to the heart can also result in angina, producing chest pains with even the slightest exertion. With CoQ10 supplementation, angina patients have been able to increase their endurance in treadmill tests without discomfort (Kamikawa).

COQ10 Reduces Blood Pressure!

Individuals with high blood pressure may also benefit from CoQ10. CoQ10 supplementation seems to help correct a metabolic abnormality thus having a favorable influence on blood pressure. CoQ10 seems to improve blood pressure by lowering blood cholesterol levels and stabilizing the vascular membrane via its antioxidant effect, thereby increasing blood vessel diameter and allowing for less restricted blood flow.

Dr. Yamagami, a Japanese researcher, along with Dr. Folkers, discovered that patients with high blood pressure have blood levels of CoQ10 significantly lower than controls with normal blood pressure. Some authorities report that 39% of patients with high blood pressure also experience a CoQ10 deficiency. (Murray)

While the therapeutic dosages of CoQ10 vary greatly depending on the individual and condition requiring treatment, patients supplementing just 30 to 45 mg. of CoQ10 daily for several weeks experienced significant drops in blood pressure, some even testing normal. There were no other changes made in diet or medication to obtain these results. No side effects were noted.

A 1993 study found that among 115 patients with cardiac arrhythmia and elevated blood pressure levels, 80% experienced a reduction in high blood pressure. (Langsjoen and Folkers)

Another study of 10 patients with high blood pressure who took 100 mg. of CoQ10 for 10 weeks found that the average drop in systolic blood pressure was from 161.5 to 142 mm; the diastolic dropped from 98.5 to 83 mm. (Digiesi)

Myocardial Ischemia

Myocardial ischemia (pronounced "iskeemia") refers to poor blood supply to the heart muscle. It may be due to vasoconstriction or clogged arteries due to plaque-buildup, (atherosclerosis). It is painful and causes organ dysfunction. Myocardial infarction (MI) is the medical term used to describe a heart attack or complete blockage of a heart artery, which usually results in tissue death.

Researchers at Mt. Sinai Hospital and Medical School, New York, report that CoQ10 may have beneficial effects to tissues rendered ischemic and then reperfused (the blood supply is restored). This activity, though necessary to maintain the health of the heart and the individual, causes a flood of free radicals and resulting tissue damage.

CoQ10 acts as a free radical scavenger and a membrane stabilizer. Clinical studies performed abroad and in the United States indicate that CoQ10 may be effective in treating certain patients with ischemic heart disease, toxin-induced cardiotoxicity, and other cardiovascular-related problems. The researchers stated that "the most intriguing property of CoQ is its potential to protect and preserve ischemic myocardium during surgery." (Greenberg)

Cardiomyopathy

Cardiomyopathy is a devastating heart ailment in which there are life-threatening heart-muscle obstructions. Usually the only hope for patients is a heart transplant which has its own risks. (To complicate things, there are always too few hearts available for the many candidates.)

Cardiologist Peter H. Langsjoen, of the Scott and White Clinic in Temple, Texas, found that cardiomyopathy patients waiting for a heart for transplant, who were taking CoQ10 for 12 weeks, experienced "remarkable clinical improvement."

Findings reported by Dr. Langsjoen, in a double-blind, cross-over study of 19 cardiomyopathy patients in *Proceedings of the National Academy of Sciences*, stated that every patient showed increased volume of blood pumped, a sharp improvement of heart strength and diminished shortness of breath.

Another study involving Dr. Langsjoen, published in 1994, conducted at the Institute for Biomedical Research, University of Texas at Austin, followed 424 patients from 1985 through 1993, adding CoQ10 (average dose, 225 mg./day by mouth) as an adjunct to their regular regimen.

Of the 424 patients, 58% improved moderately and 28% improved significantly. Before supplementation, most patients were taking one to five cardiac drugs. During this study, overall medication requirements dropped substantially. Forty-three percent were able to stop taking one to three heart drugs. They also observed a highly significant improvement in left ventricular wall thickness and diastolic function (blood pressure). (Langsjoen)

CoQ10 Lowers Cholesterol

The relationship between CoQ10 and cholesterol is not entirely clear. An as antioxidant CoQ10 has shown to protect LDL cholesterol from oxidation and studies have also shown that it seems to reduce LDL (the so-called "bad cholesterol") and increase HDL (the "good" cholesterol).

In one study, 10 patients took 100 mg. of CoQ10 for 10 weeks. Cholesterol levels dropped from 227 to 204 mg./dl. (Digiesi)

In 1994, Italian research linked CoQ10 supplementation to significant decreases in total cholesterol levels and increases in serum high-density-lipoprotein (HDL) cholesterol levels and decreases in systolic and diastolic blood pressure, in 26 patients with essential hypertension. (Diziesi)

A double blind placebo-controlled trial among patients with acute coronary artery disease with 60 mg. QGel® CoQ10, twice a day, after 28 days showed a significant reduction (22.6%) in lipoprotein(a), a risk factor of premature coronary artery disease. HDL (good) cholesterol levels significantly increased, while blood glucose, and LDL (bad) cholesterol showed a significant reduction. There was also evidence of an overall reduction in oxidative stress. (Singh)

Dosage Information

CoQ10 supplements would hopefully reduce the need for other heart medicines, such as digitalis, diuretics, blood pressure medication and other drugs used to treat cardiac problems. An addition of CoQ10 may also decrease the necessary dosage of other medicines.

Since everyone is unique, it's difficult to give dosage recommendations that would apply to everyone. With your physicians consent, consider starting at 50 mg. a day, and gradually increasing this dose over the next few weeks to the desired clinical effect. Some individuals may temporarily need as a dose as high as 300 mg. (dry form).

CoQ10 and the Immune System

The immune system needs to be strong in order to fight off illness of any kind whether it be the common cold or a malignant tumor. We become susceptible to illness when the immune system is weak. Also, strengthening the immune system is often the first step in treating chronic infections, arthritis, cancer, and other degenerative diseases. To either prevent or treat health problems, the immune system needs a strong supply of energy from CoQ10 and ATP.

Maintaining a high level of energy in the body is crucial for a healthy body. When your body is lacking energy, you not only feel tired, you also have more difficulty fighting off illness. The energy you need to keep itself running properly is the same energy it needs for an optimal functioning immune system - and it all is tied in to optimal CoQ10 levels.

As we grow older, the immune system slows down, which is one of the main reasons we become more susceptible to health problems. We become more susceptible to infection and degenerative disease as well.

Emile Bliznakov, director of the Lupus Research Institute in Ridgefield, CT., and author of *The Miracle Nutrient Coenzyme Q10* (Bantam Books, 1987), showed in his research on laboratory animals that CoQ10 has a powerful influence on the immune system. In one study, he showed CoQ10 doubled the immune system's effectiveness in clearing harmful bacteria from the bloodstream. In another study, CoQ10 doubled the ability of the immune system to make antibodies. CoQ10 even enhanced the immune function to resist and subdue many different viruses. (Bliznakov)

A study in elderly mice revealed that suppression of the immune system was associated with depressed levels of CoQ10 in the thymus tissue. This is where T-cells are produced. These are very important components of our defense system.

Studies show that patients with cancer, cardiovascular ailments and diabetes experience a significant increase in the blood level of immunoglobulin G (IgG) within 3 to 12 weeks of CoQ10 supplementation demonstrating an increase in immune system capability. IgG is an important aspect of the immune system as it enhances phagocytosis to neutralize toxins in the body. IgG makes up approximately 80-85% of the total antibody serum. Phagocytosis is the process by which some white blood cells help fight off bacteria, eat and get rid off small invaders and cell waste.

Research involving CoQ10 and the immune system has revealed a number of interesting findings:

● CoQ10 levels are depressed in individuals with cancer and other degenerative diseases compared to age-matched controls. (Folkers, 1991)

● Patients with AIDS showed a "striking" clinical response to therapy with CoQ10, strongly suggesting a CoQ10 deficiency. (Folkers) It is also interesting to note that HIV-positive individuals without symptoms had much higher COQ10 levels compared to individuals with full-blown AIDS and their CoQ10 levels were somewhat higher than those individuals with AIDS-related complex.

● The killing activity of macrophages increases with CoQ10 supplementation. Macrophages are "killer white blood cells" that combat a variety of invaders - bacteria, viruses and environmental toxins (insecticides, cigarette smoke, etc.). (Mayer, Saiki)

- CoQ10 significantly increased the levels of IgG in AIDS patients (Folkers) and in chronically ill patients (supplementing 60 mg. CoQ10 daily). (Folkers)

- CoQ10 (200 mg. daily) increased T-cell immunity and/ or symptomatic improvement in individuals with AIDS or AIDS-related complex. (Folkers)

- A virus was found to cause a deficiency of CoQ9, and likely CoQ10 as well.

Vitamin B-6 May Enhance Immune Effects of CoQ10

Karl Folkers showed that CoQ10 may have an even stronger effect on the immune system when administered with Vitamin B-6 (pyridoxine). The blood levels of CoQ10 increased more when CoQ10 and B-6 were administered together and when CoQ10 was given alone.

The blood levels of IgG and T4-lymphocytes increased to a greater extent when CoQ10 and pyridoxine (B-6) were administered together compared to when CoQ10 was administered alone. Increases in IgG and T4-lymphocytes with CoQ10 and Vitamin B-6 supplementation is very important for individuals with AIDS, other infectious diseases, cancer and other health problems. (Folkers)

CoQ10 and Cancer

One of the major contributors to cancer development is oxidative stress and the damage it can cause. Free radicals not only weaken our immune system, they can directly damage the genetic material of our cells leading to mutations and tumor growth, Because of its immune-enhancing and antioxidant effects, CoQ10 has been successfully used in treating cancer.

Dr. Folkers also suggests that as cancer is based upon the rapid growth of mutated cells, CoQ10's key role is in its involvement in the genetic pathways of our cells. CoQ10 level deficiencies are prevalent among individuals with cancer. (Folkers, 1991, 1996, and 1997)

CoQ10 is also beneficial for people taking chemotherapy drugs, such as adriamycin, that have been known to cause heart toxicity.

CoQ10 Deficiency Prevalent Among Cancer Patients

In 1991, Dr. Folkers demonstrated that the incidence of low CoQ10 levels was more prevalent among cancer patients than their age-matched controls. He found none of the healthy control patients had levels below 0.45 ug./ml. while 27% of the cancer patients did. (Folkers, Ellis) This is a very low level as healthy blood levels for CoQ10 are approximately 4.5-4.9 ug./ml.

Individuals with cancer may have a serious CoQ10 deficiency according to researchers at the University of Texas at Austin. Blood levels of CoQ10 in 116 cancer patients reveal an incidence of 23.1% of patients with breast cancer whose blood levels were below 0.5 microg./ml. The incidence of breast cancer cases with levels below 0.6 microg./ml. was 38.5%. (Folkers, 1997)

Patients with myeloma showed a mean blood level of 0.67 microg./ml. CoQ10 blood levels below 0.7 microg./ml. for these 15 cases of myeloma was 53.3%. Only 24.5% of healthy individuals had CoQ10 levels below 0.7 microg./ml. (Folkers)

Researchers at the University of Texas, Austin, also report 10 cases of cancer patients being supported by CoQ10 therapy, which has increased survival for 5-15 years, with no significant side effects. (Folkers)

Folkers suggested that there may be a connection between vitamin deficiencies required for CoQ10 production and cancer resulting from DNA damage. CoQ10 is produced in the body from tyrosine and the involvement of eight vitamin coenzymes. Three of these eight vitamins (B6, niacin and folic acid) are indispensable in the biosynthesis of the four bases (thymidine, guanine, adenine and cytosine) of DNA. Deficiencies of one or more of the three vitamins required for DNA are known to cause abnormal pairing of the four bases, which can then result in mutations and the diversity of cancer. (Folkers, 1996)

Breast Cancer

Researchers in Denmark gave antioxidants (beta-carotene, Vitamins C and E and selenium), fatty acids and 90 mg. of CoQ10 daily to 32 breast cancer patients. Six of the 32 patients showed partial tumor regression.

In one of these six cases, the dosage of CoQ10 was increased to 390 mg. After one month, the tumor was no longer palpable. In another month, mammography confirmed the absence of the tumor.

In the first year of therapy, only 90 mg. of CoQ10 was given and the size of the tumor stabilized at 1.5 to 2 cm. The dose was then increased to 390 mg. In two to three months, the tumor regressed. The researchers said, *"Regression of a tumor of 1.5 to 2 cm. in size in up to 3* months on a dosage of 390 mg. of CoQ10, but not in 1 year on 90 mg. in the same protocol, indicates that CoQ10 was dominant in the complete regression of the cancer; and above any benefit from the other nutritional supplements."

The lead author of the article wrote, "For 35 years, I have treated about 200 patients a year with breast cancer, and have never seen a spontaneous regression of a 1.5 to 2 cm. breast tumor, and have never seen a comparable regression on any conventional anti-tumor therapy." (Lockwood)

While more studies are needed, this study is encouraging. If you have breast cancer, the addition of CoQ10 (at a fairly high dosage, such as 400 mg. daily) and other antioxidants may be of great benefit.

CoQ10 Helps Prevent/Repair Organ Damage from Chemotherapy

Two groups of children with acute lymphoblastic leukemia or nonHodgkin's lymphoma were treated with anthracycline chemotherapeutic drugs. These drugs are known to cause damage to the heart, possibly caused by free radicals. The first group of 10 patients received 100 mg. of CoQ10 twice daily, while the second group of 10 patients did not. The CoQ10 protected the heart from damage. (Iarussi) The researchers concluded that CoQ10 given to patients with malignancy during anthracycline therapy is effective and advisable to protect heart function from toxicity.

Not all chemotherapeutic drugs damage the heart. Many may be harmful to other organs. For example, cisplatinum can damage the kidneys. Your physician should hopefully advise you if your chemotherapy drugs are damaging to the heart or other organs. Or, look them up yourself in a PDR (Physician's Desk Reference) or Drug Facts book.

CoQ10 and the Brain

As noted in the chart on page 8, the brain tissue contains a significant level of CoQ10 at 13.4 mcg. per gram. The prevalent existence of CoQ10 in the central nervous system suggests the potential usefulness of supplemental CoQ10 in the treatment of neurodegenerative diseases.

The Proceeding of the National Academy of Sciences reports that CoQ10 supplementation, which increases brain mitochondrial concentrations, is neuroprotective.

In a study at Massachusetts General Hospital and Harvard Medical School, Boston, MA, oral administration of CoQ10 in 12-month-old rats, resulted in significant increases in CoQ10 in the mitochondria in the cerebral cortex. It also markedly decreased damaged cells produced by administration of a known toxic substance. The CoQ10 also significantly increased the life span of the animals. (Matthews)

There are a number of conditions affecting the brain and nervous system that may benefit from CoQ10. For example, Carter, a 42 year old male suffering from Motor Neuron Disease, was experiencing muscle wasting, and deterioration of his strength. Within 4 weeks, he responded to CoQ10 Q-Gel®, two 30 mg. caps, three times a day. After 12 weeks, his power was restored. (Singh)

The term Motor Neuron Disease can include a number of conditions. Lou Gehrig's Disease (ALS), for example, is a form of Motor Neuron Disease. In this case. the nerves that control muscular activity in the brain and spinal cord degenerate for unknown reasons. The result is weakness and muscle atrophy (wasting).

A related condition which could also possible benefit from CoQ10 is Multiple Sclerosis (MS), where the nerve protector, the myelin sheath, deteriorates. Individuals with MS have demonstrated depressed serum

CoQ10 levels and depressed CoQ10 biosynthesis. (Steen)

Another condition is Alzheimer's Disease, where nerve cells in the brain deteriorate and die. Researchers also report depressed CoQ10 levels in individuals with Alzheimer's. (Edlund) Studies have shown that antioxidants such as Vitamin E are neuroprotective in individuals with Alzheimer's, but there are no published studies involving supplemental CoQ10 and this degenerative condition.

We know that many of the degenerative conditions associated with the brain are associated with free radical damage to the neural tissues. Increasing concentrations of antioxidants (such as CoQ10) has proven to be protective and beneficial.

Parkinson's Disease

Parkinson's is a brain disorder that causes muscle tremors, stiffness, and weakness. It is caused by degeneration to nerve cells with the basal ganglia in the brain. At least some of this degeneration is believed to be caused by free radical damage.

CoQ10 may be of benefit in part because of its ability to prevent free radical damage, but also researchers have shown that CoQ10 levels correlate with the activities in mitochondria from parkinsonian and nonparkinson subjects. The energy-producing activities in platelet mitochondria are reduced in patients with early, untreated Parkinson's. CoQ10 is the electron acceptor for these energy-producing activities. They found that the CoQ10 level was significantly lower in mitochondria from Parkinson's patients than in mitochondria from age- and sex-matched control subjects and that CoQ10 levels and the mitochondrial activities were significantly correlated. (Shultz)

Researchers at the Department of Neurosciences, University of California, San Diego, in La Jolla, reported that oral CoQ10 supplementation was beneficial in individuals with Parkinson's disease. Their pilot study examined the effects of three oral doses (200 mg. CoQ10 administered two to four times per day for 1 month) in 15 subjects with Parkinson's.

They found the CoQ10 caused a substantial increase in the plasma CoQ10 level. It was well tolerated. CoQ10 did not affect the motor portion of the Unified Parkinson's Disease Rating Scale. However, there was an increase in some mitochondrial activity in the subjects. (Shultz)

Note: Some researchers suggest that higher dosages of COQ10 may be needed to produce results for individuals with severe Parkinson's, from 600 to 1200 mg daily.

Huntington's Disease

Huntington's disease (also called Huntington's Chorea) is a rare, fatal, hereditary disorder resulting in death of brain cells. The symptoms are dehabilitating and include loss of muscle coordination and cognitive function and depression.

A study conducted at Massachusetts General Hospital, found that oral administration of CoQ10 significantly reduced increased concentrations of lactate in the occipital cortex of Huntington's disease patients. This again suggest that CoQ10 might be useful in treating neurodegenerative diseases. (Beal)

They also investigated whether the Huntington's disease gene mutation may produce effects on energy metabolism. They demonstrated that lactate concentrations are increased in the cerebral cortex of those with Huntington's disease compared to controls. Elevated lactic acid is commonly seen in mitochondrial diseases as explained in the next section. Treatment with CoQ10 resulted in significant decreases in cortical lactate concentrations in Huntington's patients, which reversed following withdrawal of therapy. These findings provide evidence for a generalized energy defect in Huntington's disease, and suggest a possible therapy with CoQ10. (Koroshetz)

Note: High CoQ10 doses (600 to 1,200 mg. daily) have been used in some of the studies involving Huntington's disease to obtain beneficial results. These dosage levels were found to be safe and effective with only mild side effects. (Feigin)

The National Institute of Neurological Diseases and Stroke is so convinced that CoQ10 may be beneficial for Huntington's disease that they have started a large-scale, placebo-controlled study involving CoQ10 and a new drug from Astra Merck, Racinamide. The study will involve 21 institutions across the United States. This will hopefully help increase awareness of CoQ10's benefits even before the study is completed.

CoQ10 and Mitochondrial Diseases

The organs of the body that require a lot of energy to work properly are dependent on well functioning mitochondria (the location where ATP is produced in the cell). The most energy dependent organs are the brain, heart, pancreas, skeletal muscle, kidney, endocrine glands and bone marrow. These are also the organ systems most commonly affected in mitochondrial disease.

There are from one to several hundred mitochondria in each cell and each mitochondria contains the complex protein molecules necessary to carry out energy-making chemical reactions. Mitochondria perform many functions necessary for cell metabolism, but the energy-producing pathways are the most important. These pathways allow us to break down carbohydrate, fat and protein from the diet and are the reason that we all need oxygen to live. Electrons from these food molecules are passed down a series of complex molecular pathway called the electron transport chain. The final molecule in the chain, cytochrome oxidase, passes the electrons to oxygen.

One unique feature of mitochondria is that they have their own DNA molecules, mitochondrial DNA, which carry the genetic message for several critical components of the electron transport chain.

What is a Mitochondrial Disease?

When enough mitochondria are not working correctly a disease may result. Mitochondrial diseases often involve the brain because of the tremendous energy requirement of brain cells. Mitochondrial diseases are variable in their features. The variability results from the fact that different organ systems can contain different amounts of diseased mitochondria and only those tissues with a high percentage of diseased mitochondria will be functionally impaired.

Mitochondrial diseases are whole body diseases, but the exact features of the disease vary from one individual to another. Some individuals will have predominantly brain disease or nerve disease, others will have muscle disease (mitochondrial myopathies), cardiac disease (cardiomyopathies), endocrine, renal or bone marrow disease or a mixture of these and others.

Many mitochondrial diseases result in the excessive accumulation of organic acids (such as lactic acid). These are usually normal metabolic byproducts, but when present in excess, the acidosis itself may be damaging or even life threatening. Lactic acid accumulation is a common problem in mitochondrial diseases.

Mitochondrial diseases were once thought to be rare childhood disorders. Recently it has been discovered that many common diseases such as diabetes and ischemic heart disease have, in some cases, a mitochondrial basis. Also, diseases of aging, such as Parkinson's and Alzheimer's diseases, may result in part from mitochondrial failure. In fact, the aging process itself may be due to a lifetime of damage of mitochondria from oxidative stress.

What Causes Mitochondrial Disease?

Some mitochondrial diseases are inherited. Those involving mitochondrial DNA may be inherited through the maternal side of the family. Most inherited mitochondrial diseases however, are genetic defects originating from the parents. The risk of recurrence in a sibling may be one in four.

Mitochondria can be damaged by some drugs resulting in mitochondrial disease, and it seems likely that high fat diets and perhaps environmental toxins contribute to the mitochondrial injury of old age. In the case of late onset adult mitochondria diseases, the current theory is that there are multiple contributing causes.

CoQ10 and Mitochondrial Diseases

Because of the significant role CoQ10 plays in the mitochondria, many mitochondrial diseases may benefit from CoQ10 supplementation. These conditions include:

Alpers Disease

Cytochrome C Oxidase Deficiency

Hypertrophic Cardiomyopathy

Kearns-Sayre Syndrome (KS)

Lactic Acidosis, and Stroke-like Episodes

Lactic Acidosis (As a symptom of an underlying Mitochondrial Disease)

Leigh's Disease

Lethal Infantile Mitochondrial Disease

Luft Disease

Mitochondrial Cytopathy

Mitochondrial DNA Mutations & Nuclear DNA Mutations resulting in Mitochondrial Disease

Mitochondrial Encephalomyopathy

Mitochondrial Myopathy - Congenital Myopathy

Myoclonic Epilepsy and Ragged-Red Fibre's

Myoneurogastointestinal Disorder and Encephalopathy

NADH Deficiency

Neuropathy, Ataxia and Retinitis Pigmentosa

Pearson Syndrome

Progressive External Opthalmoplegia

Pyruvate Dehydrogenase Deficiency

Respiratory Chain Disorders

Mitochondrial Aging

As we age, mitochondrial DNA accumulates mutations and deletions. DNA synthesis slows or even stops, and the mitochondria may eventually be destroyed. At intermediate stages, they divide more slowly and make defective proteins that degrade their membrane functions. The mitochondrial membranes, which contain essential enzymes and electron carriers like CoQ10 and cytochrome oxidase, begin to lose their integrity, and production of ATP becomes inefficient.

Cells can compensate somewhat for this aging phenomenon by calling for more mitochondria, and the number of mitochondria per cell does increase several fold in aging cells. Eventually, in some tissues, such as heart and brain tissues, mitochondria may not be able to supply adequate amounts of ATP, and the organ begins to fail.

Mitochondrial aging may be involved in memory loss and seems also to play a role in the dementia of Alzheimer's disease. Similarly, chronic heart failure results in part from the inability of heart-muscle mitochondria to supply the ATP needed for muscular contraction.

Supplementing Vitamin E and CoQ10 are particularly important to protect against mitochondrial aging. Both are highly soluble in lipids and therefore in cell membranes, where free radical damage is often concentrated.

Other conditions involving mitochondrial failure:

Alzheimer's Disease

Diabetes

Ischemic Heart Disease

Lou Gehrig's Disease (ALS)

Parkinson's Disease

Muscular Dystrophy

CoQ10 Beneficial for Muscular Dystrophy

Karl Folkers and colleagues performed two double-blind studies on individuals with Muscular Dystrophy, an inherited muscle disease characterized by severe progressive weakness. The blood levels of the individuals aging from 7 to 69 years, were below normal. After 3 months of CoQ10 supplementation of 100 mg. daily, the researchers noted improved physical well being, and quality of life in the majority of the individuals. (Folkers, Wolianuk)

Dr. Folkers conducted a similar study 10 years later. He concluded that while the 100 mg was low, it was effective and safe. (Folkers, Simonsen)

CoQ10 Improves Metabolic Ratios

Researchers evaluated various metabolic factors for the diagnosis and metabolic monitoring of mitochondrial encephalomyopathies. They found that after six months of CoQ10 therapy, pathological venous lactate/pyruvate ratios normalized in all patients in the study group. (Chan)

Brian, a 16-year-old boy with mitochondrial encephalomyopathy, had seizures, short stature, muscle weakness, progressive hearing loss, mental retardation and myoclonus. Following high-dose CoQ10 therapy, his serum lactate levels decreased, and a parameter of background activity on electroencephalography, was markedly improved after additional administration of the drug, idebenone. After initiation of combined CoQ10 and idebenone therapy, the clinical abnormalities did not progress for 16 months when the study ended. (Seki)

Diabetes

Diabetes mellitus involves the inability of the body to metabolize glucose (sugar), which is one of the main energy sources for the body. Excess glucose builds up in the blood stream causing a variety of health problems including neuropathy, blindness, kidney failure, impotence, heart disease and loss of limbs due to necessary amputation.

A number of researchers have demonstrated that diabetics have depressed levels of CoQ10, especially insulin-dependent diabetics. (McDonnell, Anderson) The pancreas has a higher concentration of CoQ10 compared to most other areas of the body (see page 8). CoQ10 has also demonstrated a protective effect on the beta islet function in the pancreas. The beta cells of the pancreas are highly susceptible to free radical damage. Diabetics are known to have depressed levels of CoQ10 and also another important antioxidant, Vitamin E. (Salonen)

Many of the complications of diabetes are due to free radical damage. CoQ10 and many of the other antioxidants may help prevent some of this damage.

Another reason for diabetics to supplement CoQ10 is to help maintain heart health. Diabetics have an increased risk for various cardiovascular problems, many of which CoQ10 can benefit. In addition, research also shows that diabetic individuals with very low CoQ10 levels are extremely vulnerable to death from congestive heart failure. (Anderson)

Diabetes as a mitochondrial disease

Research now shows that a significant number of adult-onset diabetics may have mitochondrial defects. The characteristic clinical features of diabetics with mitochondrial DNA mutation are progressive insulin secretory defect, neurosensory deafness and maternal inheritance, referred to as maternally inherited diabetes mellitus and deafness (MIDD). Effective conventional medical treatments to improve insulin secretory defects and reduce deafness are not available.

Researchers examining the effects of CoQ10 treatment on insulin secretory response, hearing capacity and clinical symptoms of MIDD found it to be beneficial. The 28 MIDD patients, 7 deaf subjects with impaired glucose tolerance, and 15 deaf subjects with normal glucose tolerance were treated daily orally with 150 mg. of CoQ10 for 3 years. Those in the CoQ10 group experienced improvement in insulin secretory response after 3 years as it was significantly higher than in the control group.

CoQ10 therapy prevented progressive hearing loss and improved blood lactate after exercise. CoQ10 treatment did not affect the diabetic complications. CoQ10 did not affect the insulin secretory capacity of the impaired glucose tolerance and normal glucose tolerance deaf subjects. There were no side effects during therapy. (Suzuki)

Suggested daily dosage for diabetics: 300 mg. regular CoQ10 or 120 mg. Q-Gel®, the hydrosoluble form. Also suggested for diabetics are the minerals chromium (400 mcg. daily) and magnesium (1,000 mg. daily), and the powerful antioxidant alpha lipoic acid (600 mg. daily).

Other Conditions

Because CoQ10 exists in all of the cells, tissues and systems in our bodies, numerous effects can result from deficiencies and from restoring healthy levels. The following are a few of the reported relationships involving CoQ10.

Weight Loss

CoQ10 has been shown to speed up metabolism and to contribute to weight loss. A CoQ10 deficiency may contribute to a depressed metabolic rate in the body.

Discovering that the metabolic rate is lower in fat cells than in lean cells, Bliznakov gave CoQ10 to mildly overweight and obese patients. He suggests that heavy individuals tend to have lower body levels of CoQ10 than do lean individuals. This supplementation was helpful in some cases.

CoQ10 supplementation may increase the rate at which we burn calories. One study with nine obese patients showed over half had low levels of CoQ10. Supplementing a daily diet of 650 calories with 100 mg. of CoQ10 a day for 8 to 9 weeks resulted in a 30-pound weight loss in those who were CoQ10 deficient versus a 13-pound weight loss in those who had normal CoQ10 levels. This means that those supplementing CoQ10 lost over twice as much weight as those who were not supplementing! (Biomedical and Clinical Aspects of Coenzyme Q10)

Unfortunately, not everyone supplementing CoQ10 will lose weight. If you have unsuccessfully tried many other things, it is probably worth a shot. The suggested dosage is 100 to 150 mg. daily.

Aging/Wrinkles

The skin possesses an elaborate antioxidant defense system to deal with UV-induced oxidative stress. However, excessive exposure to UV can overwhelm its antioxidant capacity, leading to free radical damage and ultimately to skin cancer, immunosuppression and premature skin aging (wrinkles, brown spots, etc.) Human aging and photoaging (development of wrinkles) may result in part due to a decline in the levels of the endogenous cellular antioxidant CoQ10 after the age of 20.

Support of this antioxidant system though transdermal delivery of the various antioxidant enzymes, such as glutathione peroxidase, catalase, and superoxide dismutase, and non-enzymatic antioxidants such as glutathione, Vitamins C, E, and beta-carotene has shown to be very effective in photoprotection. (Steenvoorden)

Dr. Udo Hoppe at the Paul Gerson Unna Skin Research Center, in Hamburg, Germany, investigated whether supplementation of the skin with topical CoQ10 had beneficial effects for the prevention of photoaging.

Measurements in excised pig skin demonstrated that CoQ10 penetrated into the viable layers of the epidermis and at low levels into the dermis. Dr. Hoppe was able to determine a reduction in oxidation in the human epidermis after topical application using a technique of weak photon emission.

Furthermore, a reduction in wrinkles following CoQ10 application was also demonstrated. CoQ10 was also able to protect against UVA-caused oxidative DNA damage. This suggests that CoQ10 is taken up by the cells and reduced to its antioxidant form, ubiquinole. Also, in these cells, CoQ10 significantly increased the synthesis of DNA and hyaluronic acid.

Hyaluronic acid is a fluid-like substance that binds cells together, lubricates tissues and joints. Hyaluronic acid is a component of healthy skin and known for its water-retaining properties, that significantly decreases with aging and in wrinkles. (Ghersetich) In Italy and other European countries, hyaluronic acid gel is injected to reduce the appearance of wrinkles. (Duranti)

These results demonstrate that CoQ10 is potentially suitable for use in a cosmetic in terms of safety and stability and has the efficacy to prevent many of the detrimental effects of photoaging. (Hoppe)

Note: Although treatments with a single antioxidant are successful against a wide variety of photo-damage, the balance between the different antioxidants in the skin is very important. Too much of a single component could disrupting the balance. The most promising study results have been obtained by combining several compounds, often resulting in synergism of the protective effects. (Steenvoorden)

Gingivitis

Another amazing contribution of CoQ10 is in preventing or correcting gingivitis, inflamed and swollen gums. Left untreated, gingivitis, an early stage of gum disease, can lead to periodontitis, an advanced infection that threatens teeth.

Barbara, at age 52, was experiencing receding gums, inflamed gingival tissues and bone loss to the extent that one of her front teeth was loose. After scraping and bone implants were unsuccessful, two separate periodontists advised her that she would lose the tooth within 6 months. She even had a bridge made in preparation.

In 1993, she began taking 120 mg. CoQ10 a day. After 5 months the front tooth was no longer loose and her gums and surrounding tissues had tightened. Six years later she still has not lost a tooth and claims she'd probably be tooth-

less without CoQ10. She now maintains her gingival health with about 50 mg. CoQ10 daily.

Gum disease generally results from a buildup of plaque, a sticky cement-like substance formed by the breakdown of sugar in the mouth and fed upon by bacteria. Plaque usually accumulates at the gum line. As the gums grow more irritated and infected, the gum line recedes, leaving pockets open around the teeth where larger plaque deposits form. At this stage, the bone that supports teeth can erode due to the gum infection. Periodontal disease increases with aging and affects up to 90% of all people over 65.

CoQ10 plays an important role in energy metabolism in gingival tissue. Various studies have shown that ingesting CoQ10 can reduce periodontal inflammation. (Folkers, 1992, McRee)

Edward G. Wilkinson, D.D.S, a periodontal specialist, reports that, by simply adding a daily supplement of CoQ10 to the diet, he was able to reverse gum disease, "sometimes in no hope cases."

Studies show that among individuals with gingivitis the frequency of CoQ10 deficiency is from 60-96%. In one double-blind study, 18 patients with periodontal disease received either 50 mg. a day of CoQ10 or a placebo. All 8 patient who received supplementation, but only 3 of the 10 who did not, showed improvement. (Biomedical and Clinical Aspects Coenzyme Q10)

Topical Application

CoQ10 applied topically (85 mg. CoQ10 per ml. of soybean oil) to inflamed gingival sites in the mouth can also improve periodontal symptoms. (Hanioka) Topical applications of CoQ10 appear to reduce bleeding and the depth of the pockets formed around teeth by receding gums.

CoQ10 can not replace the need to brush and floss

teeth regularly. Dental cleanings at least twice a year are also extremely important.

Energy/Exercise Performance

Fatigue can result from countless medical or psychological conditions. If you constantly feel tired, make sure you have a thorough medical examination to rule out any serious medical condition(s) that could account for it.

Finnish researchers examined the effect of 90 mg. per day of CoQ10 on the exercise performance of cross-country skiers. The double-blind cross-over study of 25 Finnish top-level cross-country skiers measured various aspects of physical performance, which all improved significantly with CoQ10 supplementation. During supplementation, 94% of the athletes felt that the preparation had been beneficial in improving their performance and recovery time compared to only 33% in the placebo periods. (Ylikoski)

Chronic Fatigue

Chronic Fatigue Syndrome (CFIDS) is a clinical condition in which mitochondria energy production has been implicated as a contributing factor for the reduced exercise tolerance. In a study through the Southeastern Institute of Biomedical Research, Inc., Bradenton, FL and the Institute for Biomedical Research, University of Texas, Austin, 24 CFIDS patients matched relative to age, exercise tolerance, and duration of CFIDS were divided into equal groups. Groups received either 100 or 300 mg./day for 180 days. Groups were crossed over to identical doses of placebo for another 180 days.

After 30 days, control blood and leg muscle CoQ10

levels, exercise tolerance, and post exercise recovery time were not significantly different between the CFIDS groups, but were significantly below that of normal matched controls. In 60% (7/12) of those receiving100 mg./day and 91% (11/12) of those receiving 300 mg./day) responded positively to CoQ10 therapy. Blood and tissue CoQ10 increased significantly.

After 180 days, exercise tolerance and recovery times significantly improved in both groups, but were still less than that of the normal group.

When CoQ10 therapy was stopped, blood and tissue levels of CoQ10, exercise tolerance and recovery times all returned to pre-CoQ10 treatment levels. The higher CoQ10 dosage (300 mg. daily) was more effective in the CFIDS patients. (Judy)

Note: Another important nutritional needed for ATP production is NADH (nicotinamide adenine dicucleotide). Depressed levels of NADH have also been identified in chronic fatigue. NADH, like CoQ10, levels also decline with age. Some researchers advocate the combined supplementation of CoQ10 and NADH to increase ATP productions in conditions such as chronic fatigue, and also Parkinson's and Alzheimer's. (Fallon, Beal, 1994)

Lung Diseases

Various lung diseases such as pulmonary fibrosis, bronchitis and asthma are vulnerable to CoQ10 deficiencies. The lungs are highly sensitive to free radical stress, which drains antioxidant levels. Dr. Folkers along with Swedish colleagues demonstrated that CoQ10 levels are lower in individuals with pulmonary diseases. (Karlsson)

Japanese researchers demonstrated that CoQ10 supplementation of 90 mg./day had favorable effects on muscular energy metabolism in patients with chronic lung diseases who have hypoxemia (lack of oxygen) at rest and/or during exercise. Lactic acid production was diminished and heart rate was significantly decreased. (Fugimoto)

Male Infertility

In sperm cells, the majority of CoQ10 is concentrated in the mitochondria of the midpiece (essentially the middle section of the sperm), so that the energy for movement and all other energy-dependent processes in the sperm cell also depends on the availability of CoQ10. The reduced form of CoQ10 (ubiquinol) also acts as an antioxidant, preventing lipid peroxidation in sperm membranes.

Defective sperm function in infertile men has been associated with increased lipid peroxidation and impaired function of antioxidant defenses in spermatozoa. CoQ10, as a powerful antioxidant, has shown in clinical trials to be beneficial.

In one Italian study, the CoQ10 content and free radical (hydroperoxide) levels were examined in seminal plasma and seminal fluid from 32 subjects with a history of infertility. The results showed a significant correlation between CoQ10 content and sperm count in seminal plasma. An inverse correlation between CoQ10 content and free radical levels both in seminal plasma and in seminal fluid was found.

They also found a strong correlation among sperm count, motility and CoQ10 content in seminal fluid. An inverse correlation between ubiquinol/ubiquinone ratio and percentage of abnormal morphology was also observed in total fluid.

These results suggest that CoQ10 inhibits free radical formation in seminal fluid and in seminal plasma. Since peroxidation in sperm cells is an important factor affecting male infertility, ubiquinol could assume a diagnostic and/or a therapeutic role in these patients. (lleva)

CoQ10 Benefits Individuals with Below Normal Motility and Fertilization Rates

A study at the Hadassah-Hebrew University Medical School in Jerusalem, examined the effect of CoQ10 on sperm motility and function. All 38 sperm samples had normal concentrations and morphology. Of these, 16 patients had normal motility (mean 47.5%) and 22 patients were below normal (asthenospermic).

While no significant change in motility after incubation was observed in the samples with initial normal motility, a significant increase in motility was observed in the CoQ10 subgroup of sperm that had below normal motility rates (asthenospermic).

	Controls	**After CoQ10**
Motility rate	19.1	35.7

The 17 patients with low fertilization rates were treated with oral CoQ10, 60 mg./day, for a mean of 103 days. No significant change was noted in most sperm parameters, but a significant improvement was noted in fertilization rates.

	Before	**After CoQ10 Supplementation**
Fertilization rates	10.3%	26.3%

The researchers concluded that the administration of CoQ10 may result in improvement in sperm functions in selective patients. (Lewin)

Summary

CoQ10 is a fat-soluble vitamin-like substance present in every cell of the body and serves as a coenzyme for several of the key enzymatic steps in the production of energy within the cell. It also functions as an antioxidant which is important in its clinical effects. It is naturally present in small amounts in a wide variety of foods. CoQ10 is also synthesized in all tissues and in healthy individuals normal levels are maintained both by CoQ10 intake and by the body's synthesis of CoQ10. It has no known toxicity or side effects.

CoQ10's benefits to the heart has dominated most of the attention given to this remarkable nutrient. There is a large body of impressive research supporting this important aspect of CoQ10 (significantly inhibits the oxidation of LDL cholesterol, reduces blood pressure, benefits congestive heart failure and has great implications in the treatment of ischemia and reperfusion injury as well as the potential for slowing the development of atherosclerosis), but we must not overlook its many other very important aspects.

Remember, CoQ10 is ubiquious - it occurs everywhere in the human body, not just the heart. Because of this, it has the potential to benefit us anywhere in the body and with a wide variety of health problems.

It strengthens immunity by increasing antibody levels and by enhancing the number and activity of white blood cells and other immune system components. Preliminary data from the study of AIDS patients is encouraging. End stage AIDS, like other overwhelming illnesses, has been associated with a significant deficiency in CoQ10.

CoQ10 helps prevent cancer by reducing free radical damage, protecting our genetic material, strengthening membranes. Studies have demonstrated it enhances remission in breast-cancer patients. Hopefully, more research will be done in this important area.

The antioxidant or free radical quenching properties of CoQ10 serve to greatly reduce oxidative damage to tissues. The transdermal applications for anti-aging, anti-wrinkle benefits are also very exciting. It could also help prevent one of the most common cancers today, melanoma.

We have also seen the potential for CoQ10 to benefit periodontal problems, lung disorders, neurological disorders such as Parkinson's and Huntington's Diseases, a large number of motochronidrial disorders including diabetes and Alzheimer's, chronic fatigue, male infertility, and so much more. CoQ10 even looks promising as a weight loss aid.

Significantly decreased levels of CoQ10 have been noted in a wide variety of diseases in both animal and human studies.

Recommended dosages vary according to what type of condition you are hoping to receive benefits for:

Anti-aging and preventative: as little as 30 mg. daily,
Periodontal benefits: 100 to 150 mg. daily,
Hypertension: 150 to 200 mg.,
Heart benefits: around 300 mg.,
Cancer patients: 400 to 600 mg.
HIV: around 400 mg.,
Neurological disorders: 600 to 1,200 mg. daily.

This information clearly demonstrates that CoQ10 supplementation can be very beneficial for a large number of individuals. We really have only scratched the surface of the biomedical and clinical applications of CoQ10. Hopefully, we will soon understand more clearly the full significance of this important all-round nutrient!

Bibliography

Alleva R; Tomasetti M; Bompadre S; Littarru GP; Oxidation of LDL and their subfractions: kinetic aspects and CoQ10 content. Institute of Biochemistry, University of Ancona Medical School, Italy.Mol Aspects Med 1997;18 Suppl:S105-1265.

Anderson, CB, et al; The effect of Coenzyme Q10 on blood glucose and insulin requirement in patients with insulin-dependent diabetes mellitus, Molec Aspects Med, 1997;18:s307-9.

Badmaev V; Majeed M; Comparison of Coenzyme Q10 (CoQ10) bioavailability when ingested alone and in combination with Bioperine®. Sabinsa Corporation, Piscataway, NJ.

Baggio E; et al.; Italian multicenter study on the safety and efficacy of coensyme Q10 as adjunctive therapy in heart failure. Molec Aspects Med 1994; 15: S287-294.

Beal MF; Matthews RT; Coenzyme Q10 in the central nervous system and its potential usefulness in the treatment of neurodegenerative diseases. Massachusetts General Hospital, Boston Mol Aspects Med 1997; 18 Suppl:S169-7960.

Beal, MF, et al; Coenzyme Q10 and nicotinamide block striatial lesions produced by the mitochondrial toxin malonate, Annals of Neurology, 1994;36;882-8.

Beyer RE; An analysis of the role of coenzyme Q in free radical generation and as an antioxidant. Department of Biology, University of Michigan, Ann Arbor. Biochem Cell Biol 1992 Jun; 70(6):390-403.

Biomedical and Clinical Aspects of Coenzyme Q10 1984, vol. 4.

Bliznakov, E, et al; Coenzyme Q10: Stimulents of the phagocytic activity in rats and immune response in mice, Experientia, 1970; 26;953-54.

Chan A; Reichmann H; Kogel A; Beck A; Gold R; Metabolic changes in patients with mitochondrial myopathies and effects of coenzyme Q10 therapy. Neurologische Universitatsklinik, Wurzburg. J Neurol 1998 Oct;245(10):681-512.

Chopra RK; Goldman R; Sinatra ST; Bhagavan H. Relative bioavailability of coenzyme Q10 formulations in human subjects. Tishcon Corp., Westbury, NY 11590, USA. Int J Vitam Nutr Res 1998;68(2):109-1320.

Crane FL; Sun IL; Sun EE; The essential functions of coenzyme Q. Department of Biological Sciences, Purdue University, West Lafayette. Clin Investig 1993;71(8 Suppl):S55-9.

Diebold BA; Bhagavan NV; Guillory RJ.; Influences of lovastatin administration on the respiratory burst of leukocytes and the phosphorylation potential of mitochondria in guinea pigs. John A. Burns School of Medicine, University of Hawaii, Honolulu. Biochim Biophys Acta 1994 Jul 6;1200(2):100-8.

Digiesi V, et al.; Coenzyme Q10 in essential hypertension. Mol Aspects Med. 1994;15 Suppl:s257-63.

DiMauro S; Bonilla E; Davidson M; et al; Mitochondria in neuromuscular disorders Department of Neurology, H. Houston Merritt Clinical Research Center for Muscular Dystrophy and Related Diseases,

Columbia University College of Physicians and Surgeons, Biochim Biophys Acta 1998 Aug 10;1366(1-2):199-21015,

Duranti F; Salti G; Bovani B; Calandra M; Rosati ML; Injectable hyaluronic acid gel for soft tissue augmentation. A clinical and histological study. Angio-Dermo-Surgery Center, University of Perugia School of Medicine, Italy. Dermatol Surg 1998 Dec;24(12): 1317-25.

Edlund C; et al Ubiquinone, dolichol, and cholesterol metabolism in aging and Alzheimer's disease. Biochem Cell Biol 1992 Jun;70(6):422-8.

Ernster, L. Forsmark, P.; Ubiquinol: An endogenous antioxidant in aerobic organsims, Clin Investig, 1993;71:s62.

Fallon, J. et al.; MPP+ produces progressive neuronol degeneration which is mediated by oxidative stress, Exp Neuol, 1997;144(1):193-8.

Folkers, K, et al; Evidence for a deficiency of Coenzyme Q10 in human heart disease. Int J Vitam Nutr Res, 1970;40;380-90.

Folkers, K, et al; Relevance of the biosynthesis of Coenzyme Q10 and of the four baes of DNA as a rationale for the molecular causes of cancer and a therapy, Biochem Biophy Res Commun, 1996;224(2): 358-61.

Folkers K; Ellis, L; Yang, O; et al; Vitamins and Cancer Prevention, 1991;8:103-10.

Folkers K; Osterborg A; Nylander M; Morita M Mellstedt H; Activities of vitamin Q10 in animal models and a serious deficiency inpatients with cancer. Institute for Biomedical Research, University of Texas at Austin.Biochem Biophys Res Commun, 1997 May 19;234(2):296-941.

Folkers K; Morita M; McRee J Jr.; The activities of coenzyme Q10 and vitamin B-6 for immune esponses.Institute for Biomedical Research, University of Texas, Austin Biochem Biophys Res Commun 1993 May 28;193(1):88-92.

Folkers K; Langsjoen P; Willis R; Richardson P; Xia L; Ye C; Tamagawa H; Lovastatin decreases coenzyme Q levels in humans. Proc. Natl. Acad Sci. 1990, Vol. 87, 8931-34.

Folkers K., Langsjoen P. Nara Y, et al; Biochemical deficiencies of Coenzyme Q10 in HIV-infection and exploratory treatment. Biochen Biophys Res Commun, 1988; 888--96.

Folkers K; Brown R; Judy WV; Morita M Survival of cancer patients on therapy with coenzyme Q10. University of Texas, Austin. Biochem Biophys Res Commun 1993 Apr 15;192(1):241-5.

Folkers K; Shizukuishi, S,; Takemura, K; et al; Increase in levels of IgG in serum of patients threated with coenzyme Q10, Res Commin Chem Pathol Pharmacol, 1982; 38: 335-8.

Folkers K.; Vadhanavikit S.; Mortensen S.A.; Biochemical rationale and myocardial tissue data on the effective therapy of cardiomyopathy with coenzyme Q10. 1985, In: Proc. Natl. Acad. Sci., U.S.A., vol. 82(3), pp 901-904.

Folkers K.; Wolianuk; et al; Biochemical rationale and the cardian response of patients with muscle disease to therapy with Coenzyme Q10, Proc Nalt Acad Sci, 1985; 82:4513-4516.

Folkers K.; Simonsen, R., Two successful double-blind trials with Coenzyme Q10 (Vitamin Q10) and muscular dystrophies and neurogenic atrophies, Biochem Biophys Acta., 1995;1271(1):281-6.

Feigin, A. et al; Assessment of Coenayme Q10 in pregnancy, Fetal diagn

Ther, 1996; 11(4): 264-70.

Fujimoto S; Kurihara N; Hirata K; Takeda T; Effects of coenzyme Q10 administration on pulmonary function and exercise performance in patients with chronic lung diseases. Osaka City University Medical School.Clin Investig 1993;71(8 Suppl):S162-6.

Ghersetich I; Teofoli P; Benci M; Lotti T; Ultrastructural study of hyaluronic acid before and after the use of a pulsed electromagnetic field, electrorydesis, in the treatment of wrinkles. University of Florence, Italy. Int J Dermatol 1994 Sep;33(9):661-3.

Ghersetich I; Lotti T; Campanile G; Grappone C; Dini G; Hyaluronic acid in cutaneous intrinsic aging. Department of Dermatology, University of Florence, Italy. Int J Dermatol 1994 Feb;33(2):119-22.

Greenberg. S, Frishman, W; Coenzyme Q10: A new drug for cardiovascular disease, Department of Medicine, Mt. Sinai Hospital and Medical Center, New York, New York. Clin Pharm, 1990; 30;596-608.

Greenberg SM; Frishman WH; Coenzyme Q10: a new drug for myocardial ischemia? Department of Medicine, Mt. Sinai Hospital and Medical School, New York. Med Clin North Am 1988 Jan;72(1):243-58.

Hallstrom H; Oskadlighetsbemning av coenzymeQ10 Var Foda 45:250-259.

Hanioka T; Tanaka M; Ojima Ml Shizukuishi S; Folkers K; Effect of topical applications of CoQ10on adult periodontitis. Molec Aspects Med1994;15S:241-248.

Henriksen JE; Andersen CB; Hother-Nielsen O; Vaag A; Mortensen SA; Beck-Nielsen Impact of ubiquinone (coenzyme Q10) treatment on glycaemic control, insulin requirement and well-being in patients with Type 1 diabetes mellitus. The Diabetes Research Centre, Department of Endocrinology M, Odense University Hospital,Denmark: Diabet Med 1999 Apr;16(4):312-8

Hoppe, U; CoenzymeQ10: A Cutaneous Antioxidant and Energizer, Paul Gerson Unna - Skin Research Center, Beiersdorf AG, UnnastraBe 48, D - 20245 Hamburg, Germany. First Conference of the International Coenzyme Q10 Association.

Iarussi D; Auricchiou A; Protective effect of coQ10 on anthracycline cardiotoxicity Molec Aspects Med 1994;15S:207-212.

lleva R; Scararmucci A; Mantero F; Bompadre S Leoni L; Littarru GP: The protective role of ubiquinol-10 against formation of lipid hydroperoxides in human seminal fluid. Institute of Biochemistry, University of Ancona Medical School, Italy.Mol Aspects Med 1997; 18 Suppl: S221-856.

Judy, WV; Stogsdill1, WW; Folker, K; Dose related effectivness of N CO Q10 in the treatment of Chronic Fatigue, First Conference of the International Coenzyme Q10 Association.

Kagan VE; Tyurina Y.,; Recycling and redox cycling of phenolic antioxidants. Department of Environmental and Occupational Health, University of Pittsburgh, Pennsylvania Ann N Y Acad Sci 1998 Nov 20;854:425-34.

Kaikkonen J; Nyyssonen K; Tuomainen TP; Ristonmaa U Salonen JT; Determinants of plasma coenzyme Q10 in humans. Research Institute of Public Health, University of Kuopio, Finland.FEBS Lett 1999 Jan 25;443(2):163-63.

Kalen, A., Norling, B., Appelkvist, E. L. and Dallner, G. Biochim. Biophys. Acta 1981; 926,70-78.

Kamel, M. et al,; The distribution and content of Ubiquinone in foods, Enternal J Vit. Nutr. Res.1986;(56): 57-63.

Kamikawa T, et al.; Effects of coenzyme Q10 on exercise tolerance in chronic stable angina pectoris. Am J Cardiol. 1985 Aug 1;56(4):247-51.

Karlsson J; Diamant B; Folkers K; Exercise-limiting factors in respiratory distress. Karolinska Institute, Stockholm, Sweden. Respiration 1992;59 Suppl 2:18-23.

Koroshetz WJ; Jenkins BG; Rosen BR; Beal MF; Energy metabolism defects in Huntington's disease and effects of coenzyme Q10. Neurology Service, Massachusetts General Hospital and Harvard Medical School, Boston. Ann Neurol 1997; Feb;41(2):160-546.

Langsjoen PH; Langsjoen A; Willis R; Folkers K; Treatment of hypertrophic cardiomyopathy with coenzyme Q10.: Mol Aspects Med 1997;18 Suppl:S145-51.

Langsjoen P; Langsjoen A; Willis R; Folkers K; Treatment of essential hypertension with coenzyme Q10. Institute for Biomedical Research, University of Texas at Austin Mol Aspects Med 1994;15 Suppl:S265-72.

Linnane AW; Kovalenko S; Gingold EB; The universality of bioenergetic disease. Age-associated cellular bioenergetic degradation and amelioration therapy. Ann N Y Acad Sci 1998 Nov 20;854:202-135.

Lewin A; Lavon H; The effect of coenzyme Q10 on sperm motility and function.Department of Obstetrics and Gynecology, Hadassah-Hebrew University Medical School, Jerusalem, Israel.Mol Aspects Med 1997;18 Suppl:S213-957.

Matthews RT; Yang L; Browne S; Baik M; Beal MF; Coenzyme Q10 administration increases brain mitochondrial concentrations and exerts neuroprotective effects. Neurochemistry Laboratory, Neurology Service, Massachusetts General Hospital and Harvard Medical School, Boston, MA Proc Natl Acad Sci U S A 1998 Jul 21;95(15):8892-716.

Mayer, P. et al; Differential effects of ubiquinineQ7 and ubiquinine analogs on macrophage activation and experimental infections in granulocytopenic mice, Infection, 1980;8:256-61.

McDonnell MG; Archbold GP; Plasma ubiquinol/cholesterol ratios in patients with hyperlipidaemia, those with diabetes mellitus and in patients requiring dialysis. Belfast City Hospital, N. Ireland, UK. Clin Chim Acta 1996 Sep 30;253(1-2):117-26.

Mortensen SA; Leth A; Agner E; Rohde M; Dose-related decrease of serum coenzyme Q10 during treatment with HMG- CoA reductase inhibitors.B, Mol Aspects Med 1997;18 Suppl:S137-4464.

Murray, M.; Encyclopedia of Natural Medicine, 1997 (Prima).

Noia, G. et al; Coenzyme Q10 in pregnancy. Fetal Diag Ther, 1996;11(4):264-70.

Noia, G. et al; Blood levels of Coenzyme Q10 in early phase or normal or complicated pregnancies. In Biomedical and Clinical Aspects of Coenzyme Q, Folkers, K, Yamamure Y, (editors) Amsterdam, Esevier, 1991;6:209-13.

Null, G; The Complete Guide to Health And Nutrition, (1984) Dell Publishing, NY, 474.

Palazzoni G; Pucello D; Littarru GP; Nardone L Marin AW; Romagnoli A; Coenzyme Q10 and colorectal neoplasms in aged patients. Istituto di Radiologia, Universita Cattolica del S.Cuore, Policlinico A.Gemelli, Roma, Italy. Rays 1997 Jan-Mar;22(1 Suppl):73-667.

Saiki, L, et al; Macrophage activation with ubiquinone and their related compounds in mice, Int J Vitam Nutr Res, 1983; 53;312-20.

Salonen, J, et al; Increased risk of noninsulin-dependent diabetes mellitus at low plasma Vitamin E concentrations. A 3 year follow-up study in men. BMJ,1995, 28;311:1124-7.

Seki A; Nishino I; Goto Y; Maegaki Y; Koeda T;   Mitochondrial encephalomyopathy with 15915 mutation: clinical report. Tottori University; Japan. Pediatr Neurol 1997 Sep;17(2): 161-429

Serebruany VL; Herzog WR; Atamas SP; Gurbel PA Rohde M; Mortensen SA; Folkers K; Hemostatic changes after dietary coenzyme Q10 supplementation in swine. University of Maryland Medical Center, Baltimore, J Cardiovasc Pharmacol 1996 Aug;28(2):175-81,

Shults CW; Haas RH; Passov D; Beal MF; Coenzyme Q10 levels correlate with the activities of complexes I and II/III in mitochondria from parkinsonian and nonparkinson subjects. Veterans Affairs Medical Center, San Diego, CA. Ann Neurol 1997 Aug;42(2):261-434.

Shults CW; Beal MF; Fontaine D; Nakano K; Haas RH; Absorption, tolerability, and effects on mitochondrial activity of oral coenzyme Q10 in parkinsonian patients. Department of Neurosciences, University of California, San Diego, La Jolla, Neurology 1998 Mar;50(3):793-523.

Shults CW; Haas, RH; Beal, MF; A Possible Role of Coenzyme Q10 in the etiology and treatment of Parkinson's Disease , Dept. of Neurosciences, University of Cafifornia, San Diego, La Jolla, Neurology Service, VA Health Care System, San Diego, Massachusetts Generai Hospital, Boston.

Sinatra, S; The Coenzyme Q10 Phenomenon, 1998, Keats Publishing, New Canaan, Conn.

Singh RB; Treatment.Standard plus Q gel 2caps twice daily showing relief. J of Nutr and Environ Med,UK,1999.

Singh RB; Niaz MA; Rastogi SS; Shukla PK; Thakur ASEffect of hydrosoluble coenzyme Q10 on blood pressures and insulin resistance in hypertensive patients with coronary artery disease. NKP Salve Institute of Medical Science, Nagpur, India. J Hum Hypertens 1999 Mar;13(3):203-8.

Singh RB; Niaz MA;et al, Serum Concentration of lipoprotein(a) decreses on treatment with hydrosoluble coenqyme Q10 in patients with coronary artery diseases: discovery of a new role. International Journal of Cardiology (1999) 68; 23-39.

Singh RB; Wander GS; Rastogi A; et al; Randomized, double-blind placebo-controlled trial of coenzyme Q10 in patients with acute myocardial infarction. Cardiovasc Drugs Ther 1998 Sep;12(4):347-53.

Soja AM; Mortensen SA; [Treatment of chronic cardiac insufficiency with coenzyme Q10, results of meta-analysis in controlled clinical trials] Ugeskr Laeger 1997 Dec 1;159(49):7302-827.

Steen G; Axelsson H; Bowallius M; et al Isoprenoid biosynthesis in multiple sclerosis. Molander BMActa Neurol Scand 1985 Sep;72(3):328-35.

Steenvoorden DP; van Henegouwen GM; The use of endogenous antioxidants to improve photoprotection. University of Leiden, The Netherlands. J Photochem Photobiol B 1997 Nov;41(1-2):1-10.

Thomas SR; Neuzil J; Stocker R.; Cosupplementation with coenzyme Q prevents the prooxidant effect of alpha-tocopherol and increases the resistance of LDL to transition metal-dependent oxidation initiation. Heart Research Institute, Camperdown, Sydney, NSW, Australia. Arterioscler Thromb Vasc Biol 1996 May;16(5):687-96.

Serebruany VL; Gurbel PA; Ordonez JV; Folkers K; Could coenzyme Q10 affect hemostasis by inhibiting platelet vitronectin (CD51/CD61) receptor? Heart Associates Research and Education Foundation, Baltimore, MD, Mol Aspects Med 1997;18 Suppl:S189-94

Stocker, R. et al.; Ubiquinol-10 protects human low-density lipoproteins more efficiently againsts lipid peroxidation than does a-tocopherol. Proc Natl Acad Sci USA 1991;88:1646-1650.

Suzuki Y; Taniyama M; Muramatsu T; Atsumi Y Hosokawa K; Asahina T; Shimada A; Murata C; Matsuoka K.; Diabetes mellitus associated with 3243 mitochondrial tRNA(Leu(UUR)) mutation: clinical features and coenzyme Q10 treatment. Saiseikai Central Hospital, Tokyo, Japan. Mol Aspects Med 1997;18 Suppl:S181-8.

Suzuki S; Hinokio Y; Ohtomo M; Hirai M; Hirai A Chiba M; Kasuga S; Satoh Y; Akai H; The effects of coenzyme Q10 treatment on maternally inherited diabetes mellitus and deafness, and mitochondrial DNA 3243 (A to G) mutation, Tohoku University School of Medicine, Sendai, Japan. Diabetologia 1998 May;41(5):584-818.

Syrkin AL; Kogan AKh; Drinitsina SV; et al; [The use of the antioxidant coenzyme Q10 as a cytoprotection variant in ischemic heart disease] Primenenie antioksidanta koenzima Q10 kak variant tsitoprotektsii pri ishemicheskoi bolezni serdtsa. Klin Med (Mosk) 1998;76(7):24-813.

Watts T;Coenzyme Q10 and periodontal treatment: Is there any beneficial effect? Br Dental J 1995;178;209-213.

Weber C; Jakobsen TS; Mortensen SA; Paulsen G; Holmer G.; Effect of dietary coenzyme Q10 as an antioxidant in human plasma. Medical Department B, State University Hospital (Rigshopitalet), Copenhagen, Denmark. Mol Aspects Med 1994;15 Suppl:s97-102.

Willis, RA; Folkers, K; Clinical Implications of the Correlation Between CoenzymeQ10 and Vit B-6 Status, Institute for Biomedical Research, The University of Texas at Austin, First Conference of the International Coenzyme Q10 Association.

Ylikoski T; Piirainen J; Hanninen O; Penttinen J The effect of coenzyme Q10 on the exercise performance of cross-country skiers. Vuokatti Sports Testcenter, Finland. Mol Aspects Med 1997;18 Suppl:S283-9051.

Zhuang H; Yu G; Li J; He J [The changes of PRA, ATII, ald, ET and ANP in patients with left ventricular diastolic heart failure and intervention with enalapril] Hunan Medical University, Changsha. Hunan I Ko Ta Hsueh Hsueh Pao 1997;22(4):323-68.

Index

About The Author...

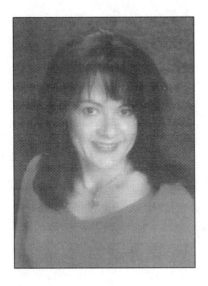

Beth M. Ley Jacobs has been a science writer specializing in health and nutrition for over 10 years. She wrote her own undergraduate degree program and graduated in Scientific and Technical Writing from North Dakota State University in 1987 (combination of Zoology and Journalism). Beth has her Masters (1997) and Doctoral degrees (1999) in Nutrition.

Beth lives in southern California. She is dedicated to God and to spreading the health message. She enjoys spending time with her Dalmatians, exercises on a regular basis, eats a vegetarian, low-fat diet and takes anti-aging supplements.

Memberships: American Academy of Anti-aging, New York Academy of Sciences, Oxygen Society.

YOU NEED TO KNOW...

THE HEALTH MESSAGE

Do you not know that you are God's temple and that God's Spirit dwells in you? If anyone destroys God's temple, God will destroy him, For God's temple is holy and that temple you are.

1 Corinthians 3:16-17

So, whether you eat or drink, or whatever you do, do all to the glory of God.

1 Corinthians 10:31

YOU NEED TO KNOW...
THE HEALTH MESSAGE

BOOKS AVAILABLE FROM BL PUBLICATIONS:

Send book order total amount plus $2 shipping by check or money order to: BL Publications, 39341 San Thomas Ct. Murrieta, CA 92562. Credit card orders: **1-877-BOOKS11**

A Diet For The Mind by Fred Chapur, 112 pages $8.95

Aspirin Alternatives: The Top Natural Pain-Relieving Analgesics
by Raymond Lombardi, D.C. , C.C.N., 160 pages $8.95

Castor Oil: Its Healing Properties by Beth Ley, 36 pages $3.95

Dr. John Willard on Catalyst Altered Water by Beth Ley, 60 pages $3.95

Coenzyme Q10: All-Around Nutrient for All-Around Health
by Beth Ley Jacobs, Ph.D., 70 pages $4.95

Colostrum: Nature's Gift to the Immune System by Beth Ley, 80 pages . $4.95

DHA: The Magnificent Marine Oil by Beth Ley Jacobs, Ph.D., 120 pages .$6.95

DHEA: Unlocking the Secrets of the Fountain of Youth- Second Edition
by Beth Ley and Richard Ash, M.D., 256 pages $14.95

Health Benefits of Probiotics
by Dr. S.K. Dash and Dr. Allan Spreen, 56 pages $4.95

How Did We Get So Fat?
by Arnold J. Susser, R.P. Ph.D., & Beth Ley, 96 pages $7.95

How to Fight Osteoporosis and Win! The Miracle of Microcrystalline Hydroxyapatite by Beth Ley, 80 pages $6.95

Marvelous Memory Boosters by Beth Ley, Ph.D., 32 pages $3.95

MSM: On Our Way Back to Health With Sulfur by Beth Ley, 40 pages $3.95

Natural Healing Handbook
by Beth Ley with foreword by Arnold J. Susser, R.P., Ph.D., 320 pages . $14.95

Nature's Road to Recovery: Nutritional Supplements for the Alcoholic and Chemical Dependent by Beth Ley Jacobs, Ph.D., 72 pages $5.95

PhytoNutrients: Medicinal Nutrients Found in Foods
by Beth Ley, 40 pages $3.95

The Potato Antioxidant: Alpha Lipoic Acid by Beth Ley, 96 pages $6.95

Vinpocetine: Revitalize Your Brain with Periwinkle Extract!
by Beth Ley, Ph.D., 48 pages $4.95

85014004R00029

Made in the USA
Middletown, DE
22 August 2018